The Original Low Carb Cookbook

Lose Weight with Healthy and Delicious Recipes for Every Day incl. 4 Weeks Weight Loss Challenge

Sarah C. Smith

ISBN - 9798671068603

TABLE OF CONTENTS

Introduction

What is a low carb diet?

A low carb diet focuses on significantly reducing the amount of carbohydrates you normally consume. As a major source of energy for the body, reducing and changing the carbs that you eat can have a positive impact on your health and result in fast weight loss. A low carb diet usually limits daily carbohydrate consumption to a maximum of 150g a day, or usually around 50-100g a day, with a focus on foods rich in protein and good fats. On a basic low carb diet, you can personalise it to your liking, as it's all about reducing your **normal** amount of carb intake, rather than a specific amount. You can adjust to whatever suits you.

How does it work?

When carbohydrates are consumed, they are turned into glucose. Glucose is a form of energy that is then carried into the body's cells, and when there is an excess of it, it can result in a rise in insulin and blood sugar levels. This in turn can also lead to weight gain when too many carbs are consumed and the excess glucose is absorbed by the body. Using a low carb diet means that once the body has burned its reserve of carbohydrates, it then turns to protein and fats instead.

What are some of the benefits?

There are multiple benefits to a low carb diet when it is undertaken properly. When you reduce your carb intake, you significantly reduce your blood sugar level and insulin level, which can be particularly beneficial for diabetic people. With no more excess glucose floating around in your blood cells, these figures will look dramatically better, which improves your overall health.

Additionally, your blood pressure and cholesterol will improve, which is critical for heart health. On top of all of these benefits, one of the biggest benefits you will notice is fast and consistent weight loss or weight maintenance, depending on how much you cut back on carbs. Much of this weight will be lost around your midsection, which can help towards a healthier heart.

Below are listed some of the other benefits you'll notice on your 28 day journey of a low carb diet, as well as how it can affect changes in your body.

Can everyone do it?

You should always consult your doctor before dramatically changing your diet and lifestyle, particularly if you have any underlying health issues. In general, a low carb diet can be good for everyone when practised correctly, and particularly beneficial for diabetics who need to maintain a low insulin level. If you do have diabetes, it's important to talk to your doctor and choose the correct type of low carb diet for your needs. If you are breastfeeding and/or have blood pressure issues, it's also important to discuss this with your doctor. If you have been advised by a medical professional to gain weight, you should consider an alternative diet or consult your physician first to strike the correct balance of foods in your diet.

Diet vs lifestyle

You may know many people that seem to constantly be on diets with little success, or success that reverses just as quickly. It's important to note that although this book includes a 28 day weight loss plan, your focus should be on maintaining a healthy lifestyle, rather than engaging in a 'quick fix' diet. As you've likely heard before, "it's a lifestyle change, not a diet", because it's true!

This book is a tool to help you get started on a low carb diet, which you can then continue in whichever way suits you and your lifestyle. As we'll go on to show you, a low carb diet has multiple results that will be beneficial to your life and will hopefully inspire you to continue after the 28 days.

Exercise and an active lifestyle

While there are no exercises detailed in this book, it's important to maintain an active lifestyle alongside your low carb diet. Getting outside is incredibly beneficial for physical and mental health, and gentle or moderate exercise several times a week - such as walking, cycling, swimming, yoga, or strength training - produces endorphins that keep your mind happy and focused. Implementing exercise in your daily life improves many other aspects of your health like sleep, focus and concentration during work, immunity and the ability to fight illness, skin condition, fitness, and maintaining a healthy weight.

Benefits of a low carb diet

Increased energy

It might seem that when you take away one of the body's largest reserves of energy, you might start feeling sluggish. In actuality, many people over-consume the amount of carbohydrates that they should be consuming, which creates an excess of glucose in the body that isn't used, and therefore you are more likely to feel sluggish and lethargic when you eat too many carbs. On a diet of much fewer carbs, your body isn't overloaded with glucose anymore, and instead turns to protein and fat for energy. You'll find as a result that you feel more energised on a day to day basis, as quickly as a couple of days into the diet.

Better sleep

An obvious side effect of having more energy during the day is usually that you sleep better at night. It can be common for people to eat late at night and indulge in a meal that is heavy and overloaded with carbs. You may find that a couple of hours later when you are in bed trying to get to sleep, you have trouble. This is because your body is still busy trying to break down all of the heavy carbs you've given it, and a horizontal position can hinder that and make you feel uncomfortable and restless.

Eating a lighter meal that is richer in protein and healthy fats means that your body is much better able to handle it and break it down, so that by the time bedtime rolls around, your body isn't still in the early stages of digestion, and is ready to wind down and rest.

Weight loss

One of the biggest reasons a low carb diet has become popular in recent years is for the rapid weight loss people notice after only a couple of weeks. Losing weight isn't all about calories and counting how many of them you consume, but focusing on what type of food you are consuming and its nutritional value. Carbohydrates shouldn't be considered 'the enemy' when it comes to a healthy diet, as there are many complex carbs that are good for the body, rather than starchy carbohydrates like fast food that are high in carbs but have few benefits in terms of providing fuel. For example, a sweet potato may have more calories than a regular potato, but its nutritional value is much higher.

Improved focus and concentration

This benefit goes hand in hand with an increase in energy. Without heavy, starchy carbohydrates to weigh you down, you'll feel more energised. This also means you'll feel a difference at work or when focusing on a task. Without needing to focus on a large amount of food to digest and break down, your brain can instead focus on a mental task. Your brain is instead fuelled by proteins and good fats, which are key to brain health and activity. You'll find that your focus and concentration are significantly improved and tasks at work become a lot easier.

A more stable appetite

It may seem that the more you eat, the more you want to eat. This is often because when you overeat, you stretch your stomach, and your capacity to eat goes up. When you reduce your intake, you may feel hungry or like you want to eat more in the beginning, which is normal and nothing to worry about. Your body will quickly get used to the new food intake and adjust accordingly, and you'll find that times when you would often snack or feel hungry in the past, your appetite has since changed.

Muscle building abilities

On a low carb diet, you are decreasing your carb intake and replacing it with protein and fat, meaning an increase in both. Protein is a fantastic resource for muscles, and you may find that if you begin an exercise or strength building regime becomes noticeably productive. Feeding your muscles with protein and fat helps them build up and repair themselves efficiently, which also reduces that achy pain you sometimes feel after an arduous session.

Examples of low carb foods

What to include

Eggs

Eggs will be one of your main ingredients in your diet, as they are very high in protein and so versatile when it comes to recipes, meals, and snacks. With less than a gram of carbohydrates and around 6 grams of protein, they are an easy and popular addition to a low carb diet. Eggs are great for satiating your appetite and giving you slow release energy.

Many people believe only the egg white, or albumen, should be consumed for protein, and the yolk left uneaten, but the yolk contains many other nutrients that are helpful for your immune system and overall health. It's true that eggs have a high cholesterol, but when eaten in moderation, they are a key part of a healthy diet

Lean meat

All meat is good for providing protein, but for a stricter low carb diet, it's best to stick to leaner meats. These are usually chicken and turkey, which are generally much lower in carbs and have a higher percentage of protein compared to products like sausages and beef burgers. Healthier alternatives can be turkey sausages and chicken burgers instead. Lamb and pork products that are unprocessed are also fine as long as they contain less than 5 percent carbohydrate. It's likely that if you're a meat eater, meat made up a large portion of your meals. You'll notice a difference in this in the recipes in this book. Meat is important for protein, but be sure not to eat too much of it.

Fatty fish and seafood

Fish and seafood are another great source of protein. If you're not a big meat eater, or perhaps you're a pescetarian, fish is a fantastic alternative. Fatty fishes that are high in omega-3 fatty acids, oil, protein, and low in carbohydrates have multiple benefits for your health. They help improve your cardiovascular health, your eyesight, and strengthen your hair, skin, and nails as well as lose weight. Examples of fatty fish are salmon, trout, herring, tuna, and mackerel. Other seafood includes prawn, oysters, clams, mussels, and if you're feeling adventurous in the kitchen, squid and octopus.

Vegetables

Just like you may think all carbs are 'bad', not all vegetables are 'good', or at least suitable for a low carb diet. As a general rule of thumb, vegetables that grow above ground are suitable, and particularly leafy greens. Try to include: broccoli, asparagus, tomatoes, courgette, cauliflower, cabbage, spinach, peppers, cucumber, cabbage, and courgette in your meals. These are all low in carbohydrates and high in fibre. Olives are also a great snack to satiate your hunger. To enhance their flavour, you can cook them in butter and add a little olive oil when used in a salad.

Cheese

High fat cheeses are relatively high in protein and can help you stay full for longer. When eaten in small or moderate portions, cheeses can be a part of a healthy diet, but don't go melting it all over your food!

Natural fats and oils

Natural fat is found in a lot of dairy products, so make sure you are buying the full-fat versions of yoghurt, cream, and butter. Greek yoghurt in particular is a good snack option for protein and fat, and can stay your appetite for a couple of hours. Make sure you stick to semi-skimmed or 2% milk, as whole milk options often contain a high amount of milk sugar. For cooking, use butter, coconut oil, and olive oil rather than low fat cooking spray.

Nuts and seeds

Nuts and seeds are high in protein and fibre and are good for keeping you full for longer. Buy unsalted nuts for a quick snack, but make sure to only have a handful at a time, it is easy to overindulge.

Fruits and berries

Lighter fruit options like apples, oranges, and pears, and particularly berries are best on a low carb diet. These can make a great snack or dessert after a meal without indulging in processed sugar.

Avocados

Avocados are a great food all around and are high in vitamins and fatty acids that are great for your hair, skin, and nails. They are a very versatile fruit and can be added to almost any meal.

What to avoid

Sugar

Apart from its natural form in fruit, sugar should be avoided as much as possible. Don't add any sugar to drinks you consume, avoid sweets, junk food, fruit juices (these contain added sugar), ice cream, donuts, and anything that is sweet that isn't the recommended fruits above.

Refined grains

These are your general carbs that you might have used before to bulk out a meal. Bread, rice, pasta, as well as cereal, wheat, barley, and rye.

Processed meat

Your meat choices should be as lean as possible, so no breaded chicken or nuggets, no sausages, meatballs, and definitely nothing that comes from a fast food place.

Starchy vegetables

These are generally vegetables that grow below ground like potatoes, sweet potatoes (see 'good carbs' below, these should be limited in amount), carrots, onions, parsnip, turnip, and beetroot. Beans and lentils also have moderate to high amounts of carb and while healthy, should also be limited.

Processed foods

Anything that has gone through a high amount of processing should be avoided. You are aiming for as many whole foods in your diet as possible.

Low fat products

Natural fats, which are mostly found in dairy products, are important in a low carb diet, so stay away from anything promoting 'low fat' ingredients. The fat in these products is usually replaced with sugar.

Vegetarian and vegan alternatives

If you eat a vegetarian diet, you are cutting out all meat and fish, which is the main source of protein. A vegan diet contains no animal products, so also eliminates eggs and dairy products. There are, however, many other options for finding protein. As a meat replacement, try tofu or tempeh, as well as a soy-based meat replacement product, which are available in most supermarkets today. Avocados can be added to most meals and, especially alongside eggs (for vegetarians), can be the meat replacement part of the meal. Fatty cheeses like cottage cheese are particularly nutritional and an easy addition to bulk out a breakfast or a smoothie for vegetarians. Beans, legumes, and chickpeas are slightly higher in carbohydrates, but also good as a protein replacement. In general, you may find you will need to increase the vegetable portion of your meals and seek out those higher in protein, like aubergine, if you are not using something like tofu, eggs, or tempeh in the dish.

Good carbs vs bad carbs

A low carb diet doesn't mean that carbohydrates are the enemy. But there is a difference between good carbs and bad carbs. Complex carbohydrates are good carbs, and these have much more nutritional value than bad, starchy carbs. Complex carbohydrates are high in fibre and contain slow release energy, meaning no spikes in blood sugar levels or feeling of sluggishness, but a consistent release of energy that will see you through the day. Examples of complex carbohydrates are: sweet potatoes, beans and legumes, whole grains, and whole fruit including its skin.

On the other hand, bad carbs are in foods that are starchy, heavy, and overly processed. These foods have little nutritional value and are broken down easily, which can lead to a sharp increase in blood sugar and sudden decrease in energy levels. Examples of bad carbs are: sugary products like cake and sweets, sugary drinks, white sugar, bread, pasta, rice, and flour, and any processed foods and junk food.

How to prepare for a low carb diet

Before you begin your 28 day low carb diet, give yourself a few days to make sure you have everything you need. The below tips can be crucial to getting a good start and motivating you to continue.

Make your shopping list

Take a look at the first week's recipes and take a shopping trip to load up on ingredients you'll need. Having this in stock will ensure that you don't do any substituting for less healthy alternatives at the last minute. Physically going into a shop and picking out these ingredients will also put you in the right frame of mind, establishing in your brain what you will be eating over the next four weeks.

Take away temptations

If you have junk food in the house, now is the time to get rid of it. Go through all of your cupboards, your fridge, and your freezer and remove anything that is not recommended in the above section. Taking away temptation is doing your future self a favour for when you are in the mood for an unhealthy snack. You don't need to throw this food away if it's still good - pack it into a basket and gift it to a friend or neighbour who will appreciate it. If you have tins of food, these can be taken to a food donation centre.

Drink plenty of water

Did you know that a lot of the time you think you are feeling hunger you are actually just dehydrated? Drinking enough water is a huge part of a healthy diet, so start drinking in the days leading up to your diet. Get in the habit of having a glass full of water by your side, and you will often find that you reach for it simply because it's there. Not only does water stop you eating when you think that you're hungry, but it can help energise you and focus during important tasks. Water is a big help for the brain and is especially important during and after a workout. The recommended amount of daily water consumption is around 6-8 glasses a day. The best way to find the right balance is by the colour of your urine; a dark yellow-brown is very dehydrated, and clear as water is over-hydrated, so aim for somewhere in between. Drinking too much water can flush out the nutrients you've consumed through the day.

Consume the right media

Seek out media that will kickstart your low carb mindset. Listen to podcasts, read books, watch short TV programmes or clips that will give you tips and inspire you to undertake your low carb diet and stick to it. If you find something that you like, this can be a useful tool to continue with during your journey.

Have an exercise plan

Decide what sort of exercise you will undertake during your four weeks. This can be anything from a daily gentle walk to a full body workout five times a week. Find out what is sustainable for you and your lifestyle and make a plan. Look online for workout inspiration, find new walks in your area you'd like to do, pump up the tyres on your bicycle, dust off your yoga mat, and make your workout clothes accessible. The important thing is to have it all ready and prepared so that when it comes time to do it, there are as few obstacles as possible.

Read up on recipes

Since a large part of the diet is cooking a multitude of new meals, it's a good idea to take a look over what you'll be doing. Some of the ingredients or even cooking methods and tools may be new to you, so getting prepared will make sure this goes as smoothly as possible.

Keep a planner

If you do have a workout schedule and a busy lifestyle, it might be a good idea to have a planner ready. You can use this to make notes of recipes, any batch cooking you want to do, workout days, gym classes, and weigh-in days. This is also a useful tool for motivation, so feel free to add in quotes and stickers that make you feel inspired when you look at it.

Take your measurements

To track your progress, make sure you take your measurements either the morning of or the night before you start. This can include your body weight, waist measurement, hip measurement, and chest measurement for a basic idea of where you are starting. Be honest!

Notice how you feel

If you're looking for more than just a weight loss programme, make a daily note of other things too. Notice your energy levels and how you feel on a day to day basis and write it down. Have you been able to get more done at work, or felt more focused during tasks? Has your ability to exercise improved and your fitness levels gone up? Do you sleep better and worry less, or feel generally happier? How do your skin, hair, and nails look?

Photo diary

If you want to catalogue your weight loss and health improvement in a concrete way, make time to take photos of yourself every day. Aim for the same time of day and use natural lighting. This may be more than just weight loss. You may notice more muscle definition, clearer skin, shinier, thicker hair, and brighter looking eyes.

Notify people

It can be a good idea to let people know that you are undertaking a new diet. Apart from your physician, make sure you tell your household members, close friends, and family about the foods you can and cannot eat for the next four weeks. This is helpful for them to know so that they avoid inviting you to events or meals that may be a threat to your diet. People you live with will be able to avoid bringing food into the house that is tempting. And of course, the more people that know, the more motivated you are to do a good job!

Going out to eat

Eating out is sometimes unavoidable, and if you find yourself in this position during the 28 days, or perhaps you are continuing the diet after the 28 days, there is still a way to enjoy a meal at a restaurant without throwing your progress out of the window.

Most restaurants can customise a meal to your liking, making it easy to switch out carbohydrates for healthier alternatives. Skip the free bread, starter, and dessert, and stick to a healthy main meal. Order a dish that contains lean meat or fish, and opt for extra vegetables in lieu of a side of potatoes or chips, or serving of rice. Opt for plain water for your drink and make sure it is topped up regularly. It can be as easy and as simple as that to maintain your diet alongside your usual social life, although you may be very tempted by your friends' choices!

RECIPES

Breakfast

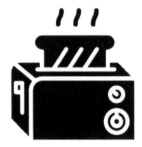

Bulletproof Coffee

Time: 5-7 minutes | 1 serving/ 1 cup
Carbohydrates: 0g/0oz | Fiber: 0g/0oz | Fat: 38g/1.3oz | Sugar: 0g/0oz
Protein: 0g/0oz) | Calories: 230-330

INGREDIENTS:

- High quality coffee beans, enough for 1 cup
- 1 cup filtered water
- 1-2 tbsp unsalted butter or ghee
- 1 tbsp coconut oil

PREPARATION:

1. Grind the coffee beans until you have enough coffee for one cup.
2. Add the coffee and water to your coffee pot, machine, or cafetiere and brew one cup.
3. Add the butter or ghee and coconut oil to your cup then pour over the coffee to melt.
4. Mix together thoroughly with a spoon or a coffee whisk to create a creamy, latte effect.
5. Enjoy and feel energized throughout your morning!

Crispy Prosciutto and Scallion Frittata

Time: 5-7 minutes | 1 serving/ 1 cup
Carbohydrates: 4g/0.14oz | Fiber: 1g/0.03oz | Fat: 34g/1.12oz | Sugar: 3g/0.10oz
Protein: 31g/1.09oz) | Calories: 441

INGREDIENTS:

- 3 tbsp olive oil
- 3 tbsp milk
- 8 large eggs
- ½ cup/ 2oz grated Parmesan
- 6 scallions, thinly sliced
- 113g/4oz prosciutto, sliced into 1-inch pieces
- 4 cups/2 bunches of rocket
- 113g/4oz goat's cheese, crumbled
- Salt
- Pepper

PREPARATION:

1. Preheat your oven to 350°F/180°C.
2. Heat 1 tbsp of oil in a pan or skillet over a medium heat.
3. Add the scallions and stir over the heat for 90 seconds
4. Add the sliced prosciutto and continue stirring for a further three to four minutes.
5. Whisk the eggs in a bowl and add in the milk, Parmesan, and a pinch of pepper.
6. Add the mixture to the pan and stir.
7. Transfer to the oven and bake for 15-20 minutes until the mixture is fluffy and browned around the edges.
8. Remove from the oven and cut into triangles.
9. Serve with a side of rocket, drizzle a little oil over the top, and add the crumbled goat's cheese.

Mushroom Omelet

Time: 17 minutes | Serves 4
Carbohydrates: 4g/0.14oz | Fiber: 1g/0.03oz | Fat: 43g/1.5oz
Protein:25g/0.9oz | Calories: 510

INGREDIENTS:

- 28g/1oz butter
- 28g/1oz shredded cheese
- 3 eggs
- 3 medium sized mushrooms
- ½ small yellow onion
- Salt
- Pepper

PREPARATION:

1. Whisk the eggs in a bowl, creating pockets of air with the fork.
2. Season with a pinch of salt and pepper.
3. Add the butter to the pan and heat until melted.
4. Add the whisked eggs to the pan.
5. Allow the mixture to spread then add the onion, mushrooms, and cheese.
6. Leave on a medium heat until the omelet and ingredients have cooked through.
7. Flip the sides of the omelet to the middle to make an envelope, then flip completely to cook on the other side for a minute.
8. Serve and enjoy!

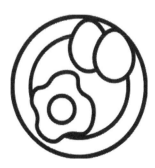

Fried eggs with broiled tomatoes

Time: 10 minutes | Serves 1
Carbohydrates: 8g/0.28oz | Fiber: 2g/0.06oz | Fat: 20g/0.7oz
Protein:6g/0.2oz | Calories: 230

INGREDIENTS:

- 1 medium tomato, cut in half
- 1 tsp olive oil
- 2 large eggs
- 1 scallion, sliced
- ½ tbsp grated Parmesan
- Salt and pepper to season

PREPARATION:

1. Turn the grill to a medium heat
2. Place the halved tomato on baking parchment and drizzle half the olive oil over it and sprinkle a little salt and pepper. Place under the grill for two to three minutes.
3. Add the remaining oil to a pan over a medium heat.
4. Add the eggs directly into the pan, cover and cook for two to four minutes, depending on preference of consistency.
5. Remove from heat and transfer to a plate.
6. Sprinkle with scallions, Parmesan, and season with salt and pepper.
7. Serve with tomato and enjoy.

Scrambled eggs and herbs

Time: 10 minutes | Serves 2-3
Carbohydrates: 1.5g/0.05oz | Fiber: 0.23g/0.01oz | Fat: 19g/0.7oz
Protein: 13g/0.46oz | Calories: 184

INGREDIENTS:

- ¾ tbsp unsalted butter
- 5 eggs
- 1 tbsp semi-skimmed milk or water
- ¼ cup chopped herbs (parsley and tarragon e.g.) including green parts of scallions
- Salt and pepper

PREPARATION:

1. Heat butter in a large nonstick pan over a medium heat.
2. In a large bowl, add the eggs, milk or water, a pinch of salt and pepper and whisk together.
3. Add to the pan and cook gently, stirring occasionally.
4. After four to five minutes, depending on your preference, add in herbs and scallions.
5. Remove from heat, transfer to plate or bowl, and enjoy.

Greek frittata

Time: 40 minutes | Serves 2
Carbohydrates: 4g/1.4oz | Fiber: 1g/0.04oz | Fat: 20g/0.7oz
Protein: 13g/0.46oz | Calories: 230

INGREDIENTS:

- 1 ½ tbsp olive oil
- 5 large eggs
- Salt and pepper
- 2 oz/56g baby spinach
- ½ pint/285ml grape tomatoes, cut in half
- 2 scallions, thinly sliced
- 8 oz/ 225g feta, crumbled

PREPARATION:

1. Heat oven to 350°F/180°C.
2. Add oil to a medium casserole dish and warm in oven for five minutes.
3. In a large bowl, add the eggs with a pinch of salt and pepper and whisk.
4. Add in the spinach, tomatoes, and scallions and mix.
5. Gently fold in the feta.
6. Remove the casserole dish from the oven and add the mixture.
7. Bake for 25-30 minutes, or until the frittata has browned around the edges and has a puffy texture. Check the middle with a knife, which should come out clean.

Pancakes with Cream and Berries

Time: 20 minutes | Serves 2
Carbohydrates: 5g/0.2oz | Fiber: 3g/0.1oz | Fat:39g/1.4oz
Protein: 13g/0.5oz | Calories: 420

INGREDIENTS:

- 1 cup whipping cream
- 2 oz/56g coconut oil
- 4 eggs
- ½ cup berries
- 7 oz/200g cottage cheese
- 1 tbsp psyllium husk powder

PREPARATION:

1. Mix the eggs, cheese, and psyllium husk powder in a bowl.
2. Heat the coconut oil in a pan over a medium heat.
3. Add the mixture to the pan and cook for a few minutes.
4. Once the edges have started to crips, gently flip the pancake and cook on the other side.
5. Transfer to a plate and add the cream and your favourite berries on top.

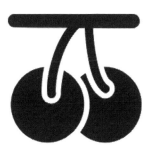

Spinach and goat cheese frittata

Time: 20 minutes | Serves 2
Carbohydrates: 4.5g/0.12oz | Fiber: 3g/0.1oz | Fat:22g/0.77oz
Protein: 12g/0.4oz | Calories: 200

INGREDIENTS:

- 1 ½ tbsp olive oil
- ½ small onion, thinly sliced
- 2 ½ oz/ 71g baby spinach
- 5 large eggs
- ½ cup goat cheese, crumbled
- ½ tbsp white wine vinegar
- 2 ½ oz/71g mixed greens

PREPARATION:

1. Heat oven to 400°F/200°C.
2. Heat 1 tbsp of olive in a non stick, oven-proof skillet over a medium heat.
3. Add the onion and a pinch of salt and pepper, stirring until browned.
4. Add the spinach and cook for one or two minutes until wilted.
5. Beat the eggs in a bowl then add to the pan, sprinkling in the crumbled goat cheese.
6. Leave to cook until the edges begin to set, around two minutes.
7. Transfer to the oven and bake for around 10 minutes, or until completely set.
8. In a large bowl, whisk together the vinegar, the remaining oil, and a pinch of salt and pepper. Add in your leafy greens and toss.
9. Once the frittata is done, serve with the salad.

Coconut Porridge

Time: 12 minutes | Serves 2
Carbohydrates: 4g/0.14oz | Fiber: 5g/0.18oz | Fat: 49g/1.8oz
Protein: 9g/0.3oz | Calories: 486

INGREDIENTS:

- 2 eggs
- 2 oz/ 56g butter
- 8 tbsp coconut cream
- 1½ tbsp coconut flour
- Ground psyllium husk powder
- 1 serving of berries
- Salt

PREPARATION:

1. Beat the eggs in a large bowl, adding a spoonful of coconut flour at a time.
2. Heat the butter in a saucepan over a medium heat.
3. Add the mixture, along with the powder and a pinch of salt.
4. Stir continuously until the mixture reaches the desired consistency.
5. Serve with the coconut cream and your choice of berries.

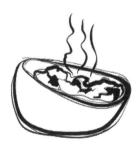

Eggocado

Time: 30 minutes | Serves 2
Carbohydrates: 9.2g/0.32oz | Fiber: 6.8g/0.24oz | Fat: 16.8g/0.6oz
Protein: 3.86g/0.14oz | Calories: 185

INGREDIENTS:

- 2 small eggs
- Juice from ¼ lemon
- 1 avocado
- Pinch of paprika
- Pinch of pepper
- Pinch of cayenne pepper
- Pinch of ground cumin

PREPARATION:

1. Preheat the oven to 420°F/220°C.
2. Cut the avocado into two halves and remove the stone carefully.
3. Slice a small amount from the underside of the avocado halves, creating a flat ledge so that they lay flat when placed with their skins down.
4. Whisk the eggs and season with a little salt and pepper.
5. Place the avocado halves on a baking tray and add the egg mixture into the middle of each.
6. Drizzle some lemon juice over the avocados and sprinkle with the spices and more salt and pepper if you wish.
7. Bake in the oven for 18-20 minutes to the desired consistency (sunny side up or well done).
8. Serve and enjoy!

Lunch

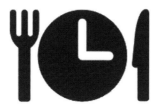

Kale stuffed portobello mushrooms

Time: 20 minutes | Serves 2
Carbohydrates: 11.6g/0.41oz | Fiber: 2.6g/0.09oz | Fat: 21.9g/0.77oz
Protein: 21.6g/0.76oz | Calories: 318

INGREDIENTS:

- 4 large portobello mushrooms
- 4 slices of cheese ie cheddar, gouda, swiss
- 1 tbsp olive oil
- 3 oz/85g fresh kale

PREPARATION:

1. Preheat the oven to 375°F/190°C.
2. Place the mushrooms on a baking sheet, bottom side up.
3. Drizzle olive oil over the mushrooms then bake for 10 minutes.
4. Remove from oven and add kale and a slice of cheese per mushroom.
5. Bake or grill for a further two or three minutes or until the cheese has melted.

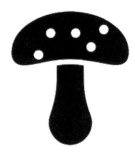

Low Carb Broccoli Cheese Soup

Time: 20 minutes | Serves 2
Carbohydrates: 9.9g/0.35oz | Fiber: 2.78g/0.1oz | Fat: 52.3g/1.84oz
Protein: 23.85g/0.84oz | Calories: 561

INGREDIENTS:

- ½ small onion, diced
- 2 cups broccoli, chopped
- ¾ cup vegetable stock
- ½ teaspoon minced garlic
- 1 ½ cups shredded cheddar cheese
- ⅓ cup double cream
- Salt and pepper to taste

PREPARATION:

1. In a large saucepan, add the stock, broccoli, garlic, and onions and cook over a medium heat for five minutes.
2. Once it reaches a low boil, cover and simmer for 10 minutes.
3. Add the double cream and continue to cook for a further five minutes.
4. Stir in the shredded cheese and cook for another minute.
5. Season with salt and pepper to desired taste.

Veggie lasagna stuffed portobello mushrooms

Time: 45 minutes | Serves 4
Carbohydrates: 13g/0.46oz | Fiber: 2.5g/0.1oz | Fat: 13g/0.46oz
Protein: 20g/0.7oz | Calories: 236

INGREDIENTS:

- 1 tsp olive oil
- 3 cloves chopped garlic
- ⅓ cup chopped onion
- ⅓ chopped red bell pepper
- 2 cups baby spinach, roughly chopped
- ¾ ricotta, skimmed
- ½ cup Parmesan
- 1 large egg
- 4 large basil leaves, chopped
- 4 large portobello mushroom
- ½ cup shredded mozzarella
- ½ cup marinara sauce
- Salt and pepper

PREPARATION:

1. Preheat your oven to 400°F/200°C.
2. Spray a baking tray with a little oil.
3. Remove the stems and gills of the mushrooms.
4. Spray the tops with oil and season with a little salt and pepper.
5. Heat the oil in a large nonstick pan over a medium heat.
6. Add the onion, garlic, red pepper, a pinch of salt and cook for three to four minutes.
7. Add the baby spinach and cook for a further minute.
8. In a medium bowl, mix together the ricotta, Parmesan, and eggs.
9. Add in the cooked vegetables, chopped basil, and mix together well.
10. Add the mixture into the mushrooms, top each with 1 tbsp marinara sauce and 2 tbsp mozzarella.
11. Bake in the oven for 20-25 minutes.
12. Remove from oven, sprinkle over the basil, and enjoy!

Grilled Buffalo chicken lettuce wraps

Time: 45 minutes | Serves 4-5
Carbohydrates: 8g/0.3oz | Fiber: 4g/0.15oz | Fat: 12g/0.42oz
Protein: 20g/0.7oz | Calories: 212 per 4 cups

INGREDIENTS:

- 3 large skinless, boneless chicken breast, cut into ½" cubes
- 15-20 lettuce cups
- 1 avocado, diced
- ¼ cup sliced green onions
- ¾ cup cherry tomatoes, halved
- ¾ red hot sauce
- ½ cup ranch dressing
- ¼ cup Buffalo sauce

PREPARATION:

1. In a large bowl, add the chicken and hot sauce and transfer to a refrigerator for 30 minutes.
2. Preheat the grill to 400°F/200°C.
3. After chilling the chicken with the sauce, transfer it to the grill for 8-10, turning over and stirring halfway through.
4. Remove from the grill and add the chicken to a bowl, then toss with Buffalo sauce.
5. Lay out the lettuce cups and fill with 2-3 pieces of chicken, 2-3 pieces of avocado, 2-3 diced tomatoes, a pinch of green onions, and drizzle over the ranch dressing.

Greek salad

Time: 10 minutes | Serves 2
Carbohydrates: 7g/0.25oz | Fiber: 1g/0.03oz | Fat: 10g/0.35oz
Protein: 2g/0.07oz | Calories: 120-160

INGREDIENTS:

- 1 cup tomato, diced
- 1 cup cucumber, diced
- ¼ cup red onion, sliced
- ⅛ cup feta, crumbled
- ⅛ cup olives, halved
- ⅛ cup Greek salad dressing OR 1 tbsp olive oil

PREPARATION:

1. Combine the ingredients in a bowl and toss with salad tongs.
2. Drizzle over the dressing or olive oil for flavour.
3. Toss again, serve and enjoy!

Dinner

Eggplant Parmesan boats

Time: 90 minutes | Serves 4
Carbohydrates: 24g/0.85oz | Fiber: 9g/0.31oz | Fat: 29g/1oz
Protein: 20g/0.7oz | Calories: 443

INGREDIENTS:

- 2 medium eggplants/ aubergine, halved lengthwise
- 1 small onion, diced
- 2 cloves garlic, chopped,
- ½ pound Italian sausage, without casings
- 2 cups marinara sauce
- ½ tbsp olive oil
- 1 cup mozzarella, shredded
- ¼ cup Parmesan, grated
- Fresh basil (optional)
- Salt and pepper to taste

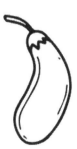

PREPARATION:

1. Preheat the oven to 400°F/200°C.
2. Scoop out the inside of the eggplant but leave around ½ inch around the sides.
3. Chop the removed eggplant and keep to the side.
4. Brush the inside of the eggplant shells with oil and roast in the oven for 10-15 minutes, or until tender. Remove from oven and set aside.
5. Heat a tsp of oil in a pan over a medium heat, then add the sausage and onion. Cook for 10 minutes, breaking up the sausage until it is cooked throughout.
6. Add the garlic and cook for a further minute.
7. Add in the eggplant that was removed from the middle and cook for six to eight minutes, or until tender.
8. Turn the oven back on to 400°F/200°C.
9. Add 1 cup of the marinara sauce and season to taste with salt and pepper. Cook until heated for around five minutes, then remove from heat.
10. Spread the remaining cup of marinara sauce over the bottom of a baking dish, then place the eggplant shells in. Fill each one with the sauce from the pan, then sprinkle with cheese and bake for 10-15 minutes, or until the cheese has melted and the sauce bubbles.
11. Remove from oven, garnish with fresh basil (optional), and serve.

For a vegetarian version of this dish, omit the sausage.

Grilled chicken with spinach and melted mozzarella

Time: 17 minutes | Serves 3
Carbohydrates: 7g/0.24oz | Fiber: 2g/0.6oz | Fat: 12g/0.42oz
Protein: 62g/2.2oz | Calories: 390 (per two pieces)

INGREDIENTS:

- 24oz/ 680g 3 large chicken breasts halved lengthwise for 6 servings
- 3 cloves garlic, crushed
- 10oz/284g frozen spinach, drained
- 3oz/85g shredded mozzarella
- ½ cup roasted red pepper, sliced
- 1 tsp olive oil
- Olive oil spray
- Salt and pepper to taste

PREPARATION:

1. Preheat the oven to 400°F/200°C.
2. Season chicken with salt and pepper then add to a lightly sprayed pan and cook for two to three minutes per side.
3. Heat the oil in a skillet over a medium heat and add the garlic, cooking for 30 seconds.
4. Add the spinach, season with salt and pepper, then cook for a few minutes until heated through.
5. On a baking tray, add the chicken slices, then divide the spinach, the peppers, and the mozzarella between six and add to each piece. Bake for about three minutes, or until melted.
6. Remove from oven, serve, and enjoy!

Balsamic chicken with roasted vegetables

Time: 30 minutes | Serves 4
Carbohydrates: 15g/0.5oz | Fiber: 4g/1.2oz | Fat: 20g/0.7oz
Protein: 48g/1.7oz | Calories: 401

INGREDIENTS:

- 8 boneless skinless chicken thighs, 4oz/112g each, trimmed of fat
- 10 medium asparagus, ends trimmed, halved
- 2 red bell peppers, sliced into strips
- 1 red onion, chopped
- ½ cup carrots, sliced lengthwise into 3" pieces
- 5oz/140g sliced mushrooms
- 2 cloves garlic, crushed
- ⅓ cup balsamic vinegar
- 2 tbsp olive oil
- 1 ½ tbsp fresh rosemary
- ½ tbsp dried oregano or thyme
- 2 leaves fresh sage, chopped
- Cooking spray
- Salt and pepper to taste

PREPARATION:

1. Preheat the oven to 425°F/220°C.
2. Season chicken with salt and pepper.
3. Combine all the ingredients in a large bowl and mix together with clean hands.
4. Spray a large baking tray with cooking oil and add everything to the pan, spreading it out into a single layer.
5. Make sure the vegetables are separate from the chicken to roast them properly.
6. Bake for 20-25 minutes, rotating the pan halfway through.
7. Once the chicken is thoroughly cooked and the vegetables are roasted and tender, remove from oven, serve, and enjoy!

Pesto zucchini noodles with grilled chicken and roasted tomatoes

Time: 25 minutes | Serves 4
Carbohydrates: 10.2g/0.4oz | Fiber: 3.3g/0.12oz | Fat: 12.3g/0.43oz
Protein: 36.1g/1.3oz | Calories: 401

INGREDIENTS:

- 2 ½ cups cherry tomatoes, halved
- 1lb/ 453g boneless skinless chicken breasts
- 4 medium zucchinis, sliced into noodles
- ½ cup basil pesto
- 1 tbsp olive oil
- Salt and pepper to taste

PREPARATION:

1. Preheat the oven to 400°F/200°C.
2. In a small bowl, toss the tomatoes in the oil, salt, and pepper.
3. Place on a baking tray and spread out into a single layer. Bake for 10-15 minutes, or until the tomatoes begin to caramelize.
4. Season the chicken with salt and pepper to taste then grill under a medium-high heat for 3-5 minutes per side. Remove from the grill, slice, and leave aside.
5. Heat the oil in a pan over a medium-high heat, then add the zucchini noodles and cook until tender, about two minutes, stirring continuously.
6. Turn off the heat, and stir in the pesto to warm it a little.
7. In a large bowl, toss the zucchini noodles, tomatoes, and chicken in the pesto.
8. Serve and enjoy!

*For a vegetarian version, omit the chicken.

Shrimp scampi and spinach salad

Time: 22 minutes | Serves 4
Carbohydrates: 4g/0.14oz | Fiber: 2g/0.07oz | Fat: 10g/0.35oz
Protein: 21g/0.7oz | Calories: 201

INGREDIENTS:

- 1lb/453g uncooked, peeled, and deveined shrimp
- 8 cups baby spinach
- 1 cup cherry tomatoes, halved
- 3 garlic cloves, crushed
- ¼ cup sliced and toasted almonds
- 2 tbsp butter
- 2 tbsp chopped parsley
- Several lemon halves
- Salt and pepper to taste
- Handful of almonds (optional)

PREPARATION:

1. Melt the butter in a large skillet over a medium heat.
2. Add the shrimp and garlic and saute for three minutes.
3. Remove from heat, add in the parsley and mix.
4. On a serving plate, arrange the tomatoes and spinach and top with the shrimp mixture.
5. Add salt, pepper, freshly squeezed lemon juice to taste. Add almonds as an optional garnish. Enjoy!

Basic low carb pizza

Time: 30 minutes | Serves 4
Carbohydrates: 5g/0.18oz | Fiber: 1g/0.03oz | Fat: 90g/3oz
Protein: 53g/1.8oz | Calories: 1043

INGREDIENTS:

- 8 eggs
- 12 oz/340g shredded mozzarella cheese
- 10 oz/283g shredded cheese of choice
- 3 oz/85g pepperoni
- 4 oz/113g leafy greens
- 6 tbsp unsweetened tomato sauce
- 8 tbsp olive oil
- 2 tsp dried oregano
- Salt and pepper

PREPARATION:

1. Preheat the oven to 400°F/200°C.
2. In a large bowl, whisk the eggs, adding in the mozzarella a little at a time.
3. Spread the batter onto a baking tray, forming two circular pizza bases or one large rectangle pizza.
4. Bake for 17 minutes then turn up the heat to 440°F/225°C.
5. Add a layer of tomato sauce, oregano, a layer of cheese, then top with pepperoni.
6. Bake again until the pizza is golden brown.
7. Serve with fresh salad.

* For a vegetarian pizza, omit or replace the pepperoni with nuts.

Keto Salmon Pie

Time: 50 minutes | Serves 4
Carbohydrates: 6g/0.2oz | Fiber: 7g/0.3oz | Fat: 101g/3.5oz
Protein: 58g/2oz | Calories: 1179

INGREDIENTS:

- 8 oz/226g smoked salmon
- 4 medium eggs
- 4¼oz/120g cream cheese
- 1¼ cups shredded cheese
- ¾ cup almond flour
- 4 tbsp coconut flour
- 4 tbsp sesame seeds
- 4 tbsp water
- 1 cup mayonnaise
- 2 tbsp dill, finely chopped
- 3 tbsp olive oil
- 1 tsp baking powder
- 1 tbsp ground psyllium husk powder
- ½ tsp onion powder
- Salt and pepper

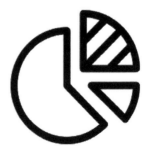

PREPARATION:

1. Preheat the oven to 350°F/175°C.

2. In a large bowl, add the almond and coconut flour, psyllium husk powder, baking powder, water, olive oil, sesame seeds, one of the eggs, and a pinch of salt. Mix thoroughly.

3. Once you have created a dough texture, transfer to a pan with a removable bottom. Using a little oil, press the dough gently to form the pie crust then bake for 12 minutes.

4. In another bowl, mix the rest of the ingredients except the salmon. Add this mixture to the inside of the pie crust after the 12 minutes.

5. Add the salmon on top and bake the pie again until it turns golden brown.

6. Allow to cool on a cake stand and serve with your choice of veggies or leafy greens.

Chicken korma

Time: 45 minutes | Serves 3
Carbohydrates: 6g/0.2oz | Fiber: 2g/0.07oz | Fat: 48g/1.7oz
Protein: 27g/1oz | Calories: 568

INGREDIENTS:

- 15 oz/425g chicken drumsticks and thighs
- 4 oz/113g Greek yogurt
- 1 red onion, thinly sliced
- 3 whole cloves
- 3 green cardamom pods
- 8 whole black peppercorns
- 1 cinnamon stick
- 1 bay leaf
- 4 tbsp ghee
- 1 star anise
- 1 tsp kashmiri red chilli powder
- 1 tsp ground cumin
- 1 tsp ground coriander seed
- 1 tsp ginger garlic paste
- ½ tsp turmeric
- ½ garam masala
- Fresh coriander for garnish (optional)
- Salt to taste

PREPARATION:

1. In a large nonstick pan, fry the onions in ghee over a medium heat until golden brown.

2. Transfer to a small bowl and mix with Greek yogurt to form a creamy paste.

3. In a large saucepan, heat the ghee over a medium heat and add the cinnamon stick, cardamom pods, peppercorns, cloves, star anise, and the bay leaf and fry until they sizzle.

4. Add the chicken drumsticks and thighs and stir in the ginger garlic paste and a pinch of salt.

5. Add in the rest of the spices and cook for 2-3 minutes.

6. Mix in the yogurt paste and a little water and stir generously.

7. Cover and cook for 12 minutes.

8. Serve with a coriander garnish and a small side of low-carb rice.

Cheese quesadillas

Time: 30 minutes | Serves 3
Carbohydrates: 5g/0.2oz | Fiber: 3g/0.1oz | Fat: 41g/1.4oz
Protein: 21g/0.75oz | Calories: 474

INGREDIENTS:

- 6 oz/170g cream cheese
- 5 oz/140g Mexican cheese
- 1 oz/28g baby spinach
- 2 egg whites
- 2 eggs
- 1 tbsp butter
- 1 tbsp coconut flour
- 1½ tsp ground psyllium husk powder
- Pinch of salt

PREPARATION:

1. Preheat the oven to 400°F/200°C.
2. In a large bowl, beat the eggs and egg white together until fluffy in texture.
3. Add in the cream cheese and continue beating.
4. In a separate bowl, mix the coconut flour, psyllium husk, and salt.
5. Add to the egg and cheese mixture, mix, then leave aside to allow to thicken.
6. Add baking parchment to a baking tray and transfer the batter, smoothing out to form a rectangular shape.
7. Bake for 10 minutes on a high shelf.
8. Once golden, remove and cut into six tortilla shapes.
9. In a nonstick skillet, melt a tab of butter over a medium heat. Add one or two pieces of tortilla at a time, top with cheese and spinach and fry until the cheese melts.
10. Serve and enjoy!

Za'atar roasted cauliflower steaks

Time: 30 minutes | Serves 4
Carbohydrates: 8.8g/0.31oz | Fiber: 3.8g/0.13oz | Fat: 5.6g/0.2oz
Protein: 3g/0.1oz | Calories: 87 per steak

INGREDIENTS:

- 1 medium cauliflower
- 1 tsp fresh lime juice
- 1 tsp za'tar
- 1 ½ tbsp olive oil
- ½ tsp sesame seeds
- Large pinch of salt and pepper

PREPARATION:

1. Preheat the oven to 400°F/200°C.
2. Remove the stem and green leaves of the cauliflower. Holding the cauliflower upright, slice downwards to create four to six 1-inch "steak" pieces.
3. In a small bowl, mix together the za-tar, olive oil, lime juice, ¼ tsp sesame seeds, salt, and pepper.
4. Brush each side of the cauliflower steaks with the mixture, coating them lightly, and leaving a little mixture in the bowl for later.
5. Heat 2 tsps of olive oil in a pan over a medium high heat and add the cauliflower steaks. Cook for 2-3 minutes each side, using the spatula to press down on each side until golden brown.
6. Transfer to a baking tray and roast for 15 minutes. The steaks should be tender but a little firm.
7. Remove from the oven, sprinkle with the rest of the sesame seeds, and drizzle with the rest of the mixture.
8. Serve with your choice of veggies, salad, or low-carb side.

Cauliflower and potato curry

vegan

Time: 30 minutes | Serves 5

Carbohydrates: 22.5g/0.8oz | Fiber: 5.9g/0.2oz | Fat: 17.2g/0.6oz

Protein: 4.7g/0.16oz | Calories: 261

INGREDIENTS:

- 1 medium head cauliflower, cut into florets
- 2 cups Irish potatoes, cubed
- ½ red onion, chopped
- 6 medium tomatoes
- 4 cloves garlic, minced
- 2 tablespoons coconut oil
- 2 tsp minced ginger
- 1 tbsp garam masala
- 3 tbsp red curry paste
- 1 tsp curry powder
- ¾ cup coconut milk
- Juice of ½ lime
- Salt and pepper to taste

PREPARATION:

1. In a large pot, melt a tbsp of coconut oil over a medium high heat.

2. Add in the cauliflower florets and potatoes, then stir for 10-12 minutes until crisp. Season to taste with salt and pepper.

3. Meanwhile, add a tbsp of coconut oil to a separate pan on medium high and add the onions and tomatoes. Add salt and pepper and stir.

4. Lower the heat to medium and allow to cook for 10 minutes, until the onions are soft and the tomato juice has released.

5. Add the ginger, garlic, curry powder, red curry paste, and garam masala and stir.

6. Add in the coconut milk and stir, then add the cauliflower and potatoes from the first pan.

7. Bring the curry to a boil, then reduce to a simmer for five minutes.

8. Season to taste, then remove from heat and squeeze half a lime over the top, stirring in gently.

9. Allow to cool and thicken slightly, then serve with your choice of side.

Tofu and veggie stir fry in sweet ginger sauce

Vegan
Time: 40 minutes | Serves 4
Carbohydrates: 16.1g/0.57oz | Fiber: 2.2g/0.8oz | Fat: 9.4g/0.3oz
Protein: 12.1g/0.43oz | Calories: 177

INGREDIENTS:

For the sauce

- 4 tbsp liquid aminos
- 2 tbsp maple syrup
- 1 tsp minced ginger
- 3-4 cloves of finely minced garlic
- 1 tbsp rice wine vinegar

For the stir fry

- 1lb/ 454g head of firm tofu, pressed
- 2 tsp coconut oil
- 2 tsp sesame oil
- 2 168g/6oz heads of broccoli, large stem removed and chopped
- 1 large carrot peeled and julienned
- 2 tsp cornstarch +2 tsp water
- Pinch of salt and pepper

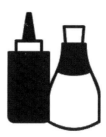

PREPARATION:

1. Stir all the sauce ingredients together in a bowl and set aside.
2. In a wok or large pan, add the coconut and sesame oil over a medium high heat.
3. Add the tofu and 2 tbsp of the sauce when the oil is hot and fry for 2-3 minutes each side, until brown. Season with salt and pepper then remove from pan and set aside.
4. In the wok or pan, add the broccoli and carrot and and toss for 1-2 minutes. Add in 2-3 tbsp of water and cover, steaming for 2 minutes.
5. Remove cover, lower heat to medium and add back in the tofu and sauce.
6. Add in the cornstarch-water mix, coating it over the mixture and allow to cook for a further three minutes.
7. Remove from the heat and serve with your choice of side.

Thai fish curry with coconut

Time: 30 minutes | Serves 4
Carbohydrates: 9g/0.3oz | Fiber: 5g/0.18oz | Fat: 75g/2.6oz
Protein: 42g/1.5oz | Calories: 880

INGREDIENTS:

- 25 oz/708g salmon
- 15 oz/425g cauliflower florets
- 14 oz/396g coconut cream
- ½ cup fresh coriander, chopped
- 1 oz/28g olive oil
- 4 tbsp butter
- 2 tbsp red curry paste
- Salt and pepper

PREPARATION:

1. Preheat the oven to 400°F/200°C and grease a baking dish.
2. Cut the salmon into small pieces then arrange on the baking dish. Season with salt and pepper and brush generously with butter.
3. In a medium bowl, combine the curry paste, coconut cream, and coriander. Mix and brush onto the salmon.
4. Bake the salmon for 20-22 minutes.
5. Meanwhile, boil the cauliflower florets in lightly salted water for 2-3 minutes or until done.
6. Serve the salmon and cauliflower and season to taste.

Vegan roasted cauliflower tofu tacos

Time: 40 minutes | Serves 8
Carbohydrates: 9g/0.3oz | Fiber: 5g/0.18oz | Fat: 75g/2.6oz
Protein: 42g/1.5oz | Calories: 166

INGREDIENTS:

- 1 medium cauliflower (florets removed)
- ½ lb/ 226g cremini mushrooms sliced
- 2 medium bell peppers, sliced
- 1 package extra-firm tofu (pressed and drained)
- 1 medium red onion, diced
- 3 garlic cloves, minced
- 1 tbsp tomato paste
- 1 tbsp vegan Worcestershire sauce
- Lettuce cups
- Mixed greens of your choice
- 1 avocado sliced
- 2 tbsp olive oil
- 2 tsp chili powder
- 1 tsp garlic powder
- 2 tsp cumin
- 1 tsp onion powder
- 2 tsp smoked paprika
- Salt and pepper to taste
- Hot sauce

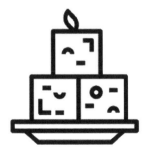

INSTRUCTIONS:

1. Preheat the oven to 400°F/200°C.
2. Arrange the florets, mushrooms, and peppers on two baking trays.
3. Drizzle 1 tbsp olive oil, and 1 tsp each: chili powder, onion powder, cumin, paprika, garlic powder, plus a pinch of salt and pepper over the vegetables. Toss to coat evenly with the spices.
4. Bake for 30 minutes or until the vegetables are tender and the cauliflower is lightly browned.
5. Meanwhile, add 1 tbsp of olive oil to a large skillet over a medium heat and add the red onion then saute for 10 minutes until they are translucent.
6. Add the garlic, tomato paste, and vegan Worcestershire sauce, stir in well, and cook for a further two minutes.
7. Once cooked, move to one side of the pan then add a block of pressed tofu, using a wooden spoon to break it up until crumbly.
8. Sprinkle 1sp each chili powder, paprika, cumin, and a pinch of salt and pepper over the tofu. Stir well to thoroughly coat, then mix the content of the pan together.
9. Reduce the heat to medium-low and cook for 10 minutes, stirring occasionally.
10. Once everything has finished cooking, create your tacos using the lettuce cups and layers of mixed greens, crumbled tofu, roasted vegetables, avocado, and hot sauce.

Spaghetti squash pasta with sun-dried tomato, garlic, and basil [vegan]

Time: 65 minutes | Serves 3
Carbohydrates: 33g/1.16oz | Fiber: 6g/0.22oz | Fat: 9g/0.32oz
Protein: 4g/0.14oz | Calories: 213

INGREDIENTS:

- 3 small spaghetti squashes
- 5 cloves garlic, thinly sliced
- 1 tbsp olive oil
- 2 tbsp fresh basil
- 1 tsp dried basil
- 1 tsp dried parsley
- 2 tbsp vegan Parmesan, crumbled
- ⅓ cup chopped sundried tomato
- Salt and pepper to taste

PREPARATION:

1. Preheat the oven to 400°F/200°C.
2. Pierce the squashes a few times then add to a baking tray and bake for 40-45 minutes. The squash is done when you can insert a knife through easily. Remove from the oven and set aside to cool for a few minutes.
3. Slice the squashes and scoop out the seeds.
4. Using a fork, create the 'spaghetti' by shredding the insides of the squashes. Scoop it out and add to a bowl.
5. Heat the olive oil in a large skillet over a medium heat and add the garlic. Cook for two minutes or until lightly golden.
6. Add the tomato, basil, and parsley and cook for another minute.
7. Add the water and mix in, then bring to a boil.
8. Add the spaghetti squash, season with salt and pepper, and toss lightly in the pan.
9. Transfer to a plate and crumble over the vegan Parmesan and fresh basil.

Vegan cauliflower hash browns
Time: 15 minutes | Makes 6 patties
Carbohydrates: 20g/0.7oz | Fat: 6g/0.21oz | Protein: 6g/0.21oz
Calories: 144 per patty

INGREDIENTS:

- ½ head cauliflower, broken into florets
- ½ onion, chopped
- ¼ cup chickpea flour
- 1 tbsp coconut oil
- 1 tbsp arrowroot starch or cornstarch
- ½ tsp garlic powder
- ½ tsp salt
- 2 tbsp water

PREPARATION:

1. Preheat the oven to 400°F/200°C.
2. Line a baking tray with baking parchment and brush lightly with oil or cooking spray.
3. Add cauliflower florets and onion to a food processor and mix until crumbly.
4. Transfer to a large bowl and add the flour, starch, garlic powder, salt, and water and stir well.
5. Once you've made a batter, divide into six equal portions and shape in patties, around 3" by 2".
6. Add the patties to the baking tray and transfer to the oven for 40 minutes, turning over halfway.

Curried devilled eggs

Time: 12 minutes | Serves 1
Carbohydrates: 0.7g/0.02oz | Fat: 10.2g/0.34oz
Protein: 5.7g/0.2oz | Calories: 120

INGREDIENTS:

- 1 medium egg
- 2 tsp mayonnaise
- ¼ tsp curry powder
- Pinch of salt

PREPARATION:

1. Put the egg in a saucepan of cold water and bring to the boil. When the water bubbles, bring to a simmer and cook for 6 minutes. Remove from pan, rinse with cold water, peel, and cut the egg in half.
2. Once cold, scoop out the yolk. Mix yolk with mayonnaise and curry powder.
3. Spoon the yolk mixture back into the cooked egg white.
4. Garnish with a little extra curry powder and enjoy.

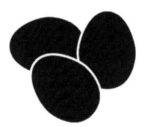

Banana waffles

Time: 10 minutes | Serves 2
Carbohydrates: 4g/0.14oz | Fiber: 2g/0.07oz | Fat: 13g/0.46oz
Protein: 5g/0.18oz | Calories: 155

INGREDIENTS:

- 1 egg
- ¼ ripe banana
- 3 tbsp coconut milk
- 3 tbsp almond flour
- ¼ tbsp ground psyllium husk powder

- ¼ tsp baking powder
- ⅛ tsp vanilla extract
- ¼ tsp ground cinnamon
- Coconut oil or butter
- Pinch of salt

PREPARATION:

1. In a large bowl, mix together all of the ingredients, adding one at a time and whisking thoroughly.
2. Fry in a frying pan or add mixture to a waffle iron.
3. Serve with your choice of side: Greek yogurt, berries, butter, or hazelnut spread.

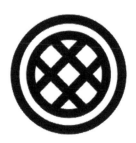

Fro-yo popsicles

Time: 20 minutes | Makes 12 popsicles
Carbohydrates: 5g/0.18oz | Fiber: 1g/0.03oz | Fat: 5g/0.18oz
Protein: 2g/0.07oz | Calories: 72

INGREDIENTS:

- 4 oz/100g frozen mango, diced
- 4 oz/100g frozen strawberries
- ½ cup Greek yogurt
- ¼ cup heavy whipping cream
- ½ tsp vanilla extract

PREPARATION:

1. Allow mango and strawberries to thaw for 10-15 minutes.
2. Add all the ingredients to a blender and mix until smooth.
3. Pour into popsicle trays and freeze for at least a couple of hours.
4. Enjoy as a quick and tasty treat!

Saffron Panna Cotta

Time: 120 minutes |Serves 6
Carbohydrates: 2g/0.07oz | Fiber: 0g/0oz | Fat: 29g/1oz
Protein: 3g/0.1oz | Calories: 270

INGREDIENTS:

- 12 raspberries
- 2 cups heavy whipping cream
- 1 tbsp chopped almonds
- 1 tbsp honey
- ½ cup water
- ½ tbsp powdered gelatin
- ¼ tsp vanilla extract
- Pinch of saffron

PREPARATION:

1. Mix the gelatin and water together.
2. In a saucepan, add the cream, vanilla, honey, and saffron and bring to a boil.
3. Reduce and simmer for 2-3 minutes, add gelatin mix and stir.
4. Transfer mixture to 6 dessert glasses and cover.
5. Refrigerate for 2-3 hours and serve with raspberries and almonds.

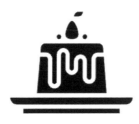

Smoothies

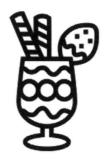

Spinach and avocado "green" smoothie

Time: 5 minutes | Serves 1
Carbohydrates: 3.5g/0.1oz | Fiber: 7g/0.25oz | Calories: 165

INGREDIENTS:

- 2 cups spinach
- ½ avocado, pitted and chopped
- 1 cup plant milk
- 1 ½ cups ice
- ¼ cup vanilla protein powder
- ¼ cup sweetener/Stevia

PREPARATION:

1. Add your choice of plant milk and spinach to a smoothie blender, then add the remaining ingredients one at a time.
2. Blend on high until completely smooth. Add milk or ice if necessary.
3. Recipe makes one serving, enjoy in a large glass or two smaller servings.

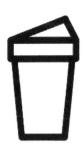

Blueberry Smoothie

Time: 5 minutes | Serves 1
Carbohydrates: 10g/0.35oz | Fiber: 1g/0.04oz | Fat: 43g/1.5oz
Protein: 4g/0.14oz | Calories: 415

INGREDIENTS:

- 7 oz/200g coconut milk
- ½ tbsp lemon juice
- ¼ cup blueberries
- ¼ tsp vanilla extract

PREPARATION:

1. Add all of the ingredients to a smoothie maker, blender, or food processor.

2. Blend together on high until the texture is smooth.

3. Pour into a glass over a couple of ice cubes and enjoy!

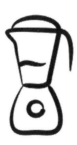

Chocolate berry smoothie

Time: 5 minutes | Serves 2
Carbohydrates: 15g/0.53oz | Fiber: 26g/0.92oz | Fat: 26g/0.92oz
Protein: 3g/0.1oz | Calories: 294

INGREDIENTS:

- ½ an avocado
- 1½ tbsp unsweetened cocoa powder
- 2g/0.07oz sweetener or stevia
- 2 tbsp pecans or almonds
- ¾ teaspoon pure vanilla extract
- ¼ cup heavy whipping cream
- ½ cup water
- ¾ cup frozen mixed berries our mix includes raspberries, strawberries, and blueberries
- ¾ cup ice cubes
- Salt
- Berries for topping (optional)

PREPARATION:

1. Add all of the ingredients, except ice, to a blender or smoothie maker and blend on high until smooth.
2. Stir through to check consistency then add the ice and pulse until smooth.
3. Transfer to a glass and add your desired toppings
4. Enjoy!

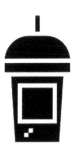

28 DAY WEIGHT LOSS PLAN

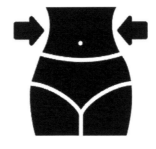

DAY 1

Breakfast: Scrambled eggs and herbs (See page 33)

Lunch: Broccoli and cheese omelet
Time: 5 minutes | Serves 1
Carbohydrates: 6.4g/0.26oz | Fiber: 2.6g/0.1oz | Fat: 8.5g/0.3oz
Protein: 20.6g/0.73oz | Calories: 184

INGREDIENTS:

- 1 egg
- 2 egg whites
- 1 tbsp milk
- Salt and pepper
- Oil for cooking
- ½ cup broccoli, cooked
- 1 slice Swiss cheese

PREPARATION:

1. In a small bowl, add the egg, egg whites, milk, salt and pepper and beat until smooth.
2. Spray a medium nonstick skillet with cooking spray and place over a medium heat.
3. Add the eggs mixture to the pan, cook for a minute then reduce the heat.
4. Add the cheese and broccoli.
5. Once the omelet is set, flip the sides into the middle.

Dinner: Za'atar roasted cauliflower steaks (See page 59)

DAY 2

Breakfast: Greek frittata (See page 34)

Lunch: Kale stuffed portobello mushrooms (See page 40)

Dinner: Chicken broccoli with dill sauce
Time: 30 minutes | Serves 4
Net carbs: 6g/0.2oz | Fiber: 2g/0.07oz | Fat: 9g/0.3oz
Protein: 39g/1.38oz | Calories: 274

INGREDIENTS:

- 4 6oz/170g skinless boneless chicken breast halves
- 1 cup milk
- 4 cups broccoli florets
- 1 tbsp all-purpose flour
- 1 cup chicken stock
- 1 tbsp fresh dill
- 1 tbsp olive oil
- ½ tsp garlic salt
- ¼ tsp pepper

PREPARATION:

1. Add the chicken to a pan over a medium heat and season with pepper and garlic salt. Cook gently until it browns.
2. Remove the chicken from the pan and add the broccoli and stock. Bring to a boil then simmer for 5 minutes.
3. In a bowl, add the flour, dill, and milk, and stir. Add to the pan with the broccoli and cook until it thickens.
4. Re-introduce the chicken and cook until fully cooked through.
5. Transfer to a plate or bowl and serve.

DAY 3

Breakfast: Eggocado (See page 38)

Lunch: Goat cheese salad with balsamic butter
Time: 15 minutes | Serves 2
Carbohydrates: 3g/0.1oz | Fiber: 2g/0.07oz | Fat: 73g/2.6oz
Protein: 37g/1.3oz | Calories: 824

INGREDIENTS:

- 10 oz/ 283g sliced goat cheese
- 3 oz/85g baby spinach
- 2 oz/ 57g butter
- ¼ cup pumpkin seeds
- 1 tbsp balsamic vinegar

PREPARATION:

1. Preheat oven to 400°F/200°C
2. Bake cheese slices on a baking tray for 10 minutes.
3. Toast pumpkin seeds until they pop.
4. Reduce the temperature, add butter, then bake until golden brown.
5. Add vinegar and boil for 5 minutes.
6. Serve with spinach.

Dinner: Thai fish curry with coconut (See page 64)

DAY 4

Breakfast: Pancakes with cream and berries (See page 35)

Lunch: Greek salad (See page 45)

Dinner: Turkey with cream cheese sauce
Time: 25 minutes | Serves 4
Net carbs: 7g/0.3oz | Fiber: 0g/0oz | Fat: 67g/2.4oz
Protein: 43g/1.5oz | Calories: 793

INGREDIENTS:

- 20 oz/566g turkey breast
- 7 oz/200g cream cheese
- 2 cups double cream
- ⅓ cup small capers
- 1 tbsp tamari soy sauce
- 2 tbsp butter
- Salt and pepper

PREPARATION:

1. Preheat the oven to 350°F/175°C.
2. Heat 1 tbsp butter in an ovenproof frying pan. Season the turkey and add it to the pan, frying until golden brown.
3. Transfer the pan to the oven for 5-6 minutes then remove and transfer to a plate.
4. Separate the turkey drippings, transfer to a pan and add the cheese and cream, stirring until it boils lightly. Reduce to a simmer, allow to thicken, and season.
5. Saute the capers with 1 tbsp butter until crisp, then serve with turkey and gravy.

DAY 5

Breakfast: Soft Tortillas

Time: 40 minutes | Serves 12
Net carbs: 2g/0.07oz | Fiber: 15g/0.5oz | Fat: 21g/0.74oz
Protein: 6g/0.25oz | Calories: 250

INGREDIENTS:

- 6 large egg whites
- 3 cups hot water
- 2 cups coconut flour
- 1 cup olive oil
- ½ cup ground psyllium husk powder
- 1 tsp salt
- ½ tsp baking soda

PREPARATION:

1. In a bowl, mix baking soda, coconut flour, psyllium husk powder, and salt.
2. Add the oil a little at a time and stir.
3. Add the egg whites and a little hot water at a time, stirring in between.
4. Shape into 12 balls and press flat onto a baking tray.
5. Bake 3 minutes per side until brown.
6. Serve with your choice of toppings.

Lunch: Grilled Buffalo chicken lettuce wraps (See page 44)

Dinner: Spaghetti squash pasta with sun-dried tomato, garlic, and basil (See page 67)

DAY 6

Breakfast: Crispy prosciutto and scallion frittata (See page 30)

Lunch: Caprese Omelet
Time: 20 minutes | Serves 2
Carbohydrates: 4g/0.14oz | Fiber: 1g/0.03oz | Fat: 43g/1.5oz
Protein: 33g/1.16oz | Calories: 534

INGREDIENTS:

- 5 oz/ 141g mozzarella cheese
- 3 oz/ 85g tomatoes, sliced
- 6 eggs
- 1 tbsp basil
- 2 tbsp olive oil
- Salt and pepper

PREPARATION:

1. Beat the eggs with the seasoning and basil.
2. Fry the tomatoes for 5 minutes.
3. Add in the egg mixture, mix until firm.
4. Add the cheese, reduce the temperature.
5. When set, fold sides into the middle.

Dinner: Vegan roasted cauliflower tofu tacos (See page 65)

DAY 7

Breakfast: Mushroom omelet (See page 31)

Lunch: Skinny shrimp scampi and zoodles
Time: 27 minutes | Serves 2
Carbohydrates: 4g/0.14oz | Fiber: 4g/0.14oz | Fat: 7g/0.25oz
Protein: 11g/0.4oz | Calories: 170

INGREDIENTS:

- 3 cups zoodles
- 12 large shrimp, shelled and deveined
- 2 tbsp butter/oil
- 2 tsp garlic, minced
- 2½ tbsp white wine
- 1½ tbsp fresh lemon juice
- 2 tsp grated Parmesan

PREPARATION:

1. Microwave zoodles for 2 minutes.
2. Heat butter/oil over a medium-low heat in a large pan.
3. Add garlic and cook for 1 minute.
4. Add shrimp and cook for 2 minutes. Season then transfer to a bowl.
5. Increase heat a little, add wine and lemon juice and cook for 2 minutes.
6. Add the zoodles and shrimp and toss for 30 seconds.
7. Serve with Parmesan.

Dinner: Balsamic chicken with roast vegetables (See page 50)

DAY 8

Breakfast: Green smoothie (See page 75)

Lunch: Tuna stuffed tomatoes
Time: 25 minutes | Serves 4
Carbohydrates: 8g/0.3oz | Fiber: 2g/0.07oz | Fat: 10g/0.35oz
Protein: 13g/0.46oz | Calories: 170

INGREDIENTS:

- 8 small tomatoes
- 2 tins tuna
- 10 pitted kalamata olives, minced
- 2 tbsp fresh parsley, minced
- 1 tbsp capers
- 1 tbsp olive oil
- ½ tsp fresh thyme leaves, minced
- Salt and pepper

PREPARATION:

1. Slice the top of each tomato and scoop out the seeds and pulp.
2. Place tomato shells down on a paper towel to drain.
3. Mix tuna, olives, capers, oil, parsley, thyme, and pepper in a bowl.
4. Season with salt and pepper, then spoon into tomatoes and serve.

Dinner: Pesto zucchini noodles with grilled chicken and roasted tomatoes (See page 51)

DAY 9

Breakfast: Paleo bread
Time: 65 minutes | Serves 20
Carbohydrates: 24g/0.85oz | Fiber: 4g/0.14oz | Fat: 24g/0.85oz
Protein: 10g/0.35oz | Calories: 266

INGREDIENTS:

- 6 eggs
- 7 oz/200g pumpkin seeds
- 7 oz/200g almonds
- 4 oz/114g sunflower seeds
- 3 oz/85g sesame seeds
- 3 oz/85g flaxseed
- 2 oz/57g walnuts
- ⅓ cup olive oil
- 1 tbsp crushed fennel seeds
- 2 tsp salt
- ½ tsp white wine vinegar

PREPARATION:

1. Preheat the oven to 300°F/150°C.
2. Mix the dry ingredients in a bowl, adding the oil, eggs, and vinegar a little at a time.
3. Add the dough to a non stick bread pan and bake for an hour.
4. Serve with your choice of sides or toppings.

Lunch: Kale stuffed portobello mushrooms (See page 40)

Dinner: Thai fish curry with coconut (See page 64)

DAY 10

Breakfast: Bulletproof coffee (See page 29)

Lunch: BLT chicken salad
Time: 20 minutes | Serves 8
Carbohydrates: 5g/0.18oz | Fiber: 2g/0.07oz | Fat: 19g/0.67oz
Protein: 23g/0.481oz | Calories: 281

INGREDIENTS:

- 1½ lb/680g boneless skinless chicken breasts, cooked and cubed
- 10 bacon strips, cooked and crumbled
- 2 hard-boiled large eggs, sliced
- ½ cup mayonnaise
- 4 tbsp barbecue sauce
- 8 cups salad greens
- 2 large tomatoes, chopped
- 2 tbsp onion, finely chopped
- 1 tbsp lemon juice
- ¼ tsp pepper

PREPARATION:

1. Combine the mayonnaise, barbecue sauce, lemon juice, onion and pepper in a bowl and mix well. Cover and refrigerate.
2. Toss the salad greens, tomatoes, chicken and bacon in a bowl then garnish with eggs.
3. Drizzle with refrigerated dressing and serve.

Dinner: (See page 62)

DAY 11

Breakfast: Coconut milk strawberry smoothie
Time: 2 minutes | Serves 2
Carbohydrates: 15g/0.53oz | Fiber: 5g/0.18oz | Fat: 26g/0.92oz
Protein: 6g/0.21oz | Calories: 397

INGREDIENTS:

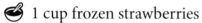 1 cup frozen strawberries   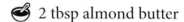 2 tbsp almond butter

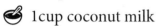 1cup coconut milk

PREPARATION:

1. Add the ingredients to a blender and process until completely smooth.
2. Pour into a glass and enjoy, adding a tsp of sweetener to taste.

Lunch: Greek salad (See page 45)

Dinner: Cauliflower and potato curry (See page 60)

DAY 12

Breakfast: Crispy prosciutto and scallion frittata (See page 30)

Lunch: Cauliflower soup
Time: 30 minutes | Serves 8
Carbohydrates: 10g/0.4oz | Fiber: 2g/0.07oz | Fat: 11g/0.4oz
Protein: 7g/0.25oz | Calories: 159

INGREDIENTS:

- 1 medium head cauliflower, broken into florets
- 1 medium carrot, shredded
- ¼ cup chopped celery
- 2 ½ cups vegetable stock
- 3 tbsp butter
- 3 tbsp all-purpose flour
- ¾ teaspoon salt
- ⅛ teaspoon pepper
- 2 cups milk
- 1 cup shredded cheddar cheese

PREPARATION:

1. Add the florets, celery, carrot, and stock to a Dutch oven and bring to a boil.
2. Reduce heat, cover, and simmer for 15 minutes.
3. Melt the butter in a large pan and add the flour and seasoning, stirring well.
4. Add in milk gradually and bring to a boil.
5. Cook for 2 minutes until thick then reduce heat and add cheese.
6. Add in the cauliflower mixture and stir.

Dinner: Chicken korma (See page 56)

DAY 13

Breakfast: Chocolate berry smoothie (See page 77)

Lunch: Fontina asparagus tart
Time: 35 minutes | Serves 8
Carbohydrates: 10g/0.4oz | Fiber: 1g/0.03oz | Fat: 9g/0.3oz
Protein: 5g/0.2oz | Calories: 142

INGREDIENTS:

- ½ lb asparagus, trimmed
- ½ sheet puff pastry
- 1 cup shredded fontina cheese
- ½ tsp grated lemon zest
- 1 tbsp lemon juice
- ½ tbsp olive oil
- Pinch of salt and pepper

PREPARATION:

1. Preheat oven to 400°F/200°C.
2. Bring ½ inch water to a boil in a large skillet then add asparagus and cover and cook for 5 minutes.
3. Drain and pat dry.
4. Roll pastry on a floured surface to a 8"x6" rectangle. Transfer to a parchment-lined baking tray and bake for 10 minutes.
5. Remove and sprinkle with half the cheese. Put the cooked asparagus on top and sprinkle remaining cheese.
6. Mix the remaining ingredients and drizzle over the pastry.
7. Bake for a further 12-15 minutes and serve.

Dinner: Za'atar roasted cauliflower steaks (See page 59)

DAY 14

Breakfast: Chocolate peanut butter smoothie

Time: 5 minutes | Serves 8

Carbohydrates: 11g/0.4oz | Fiber: 5g/0.15oz | Fat:33g/1.17oz

Protein: 7g/0.25oz | Calories: 352

INGREDIENTS:

- 1 tbsp 100% peanut butter
- ¼ cup double cream
- 1 tsp vanilla extract
- ¼ tsp espresso powder
- ½ cup water
- 1 tbsp cocoa powder
- ½ tbsp chia seeds
- 12 drops liquid stevia
- 1 pinch sea salt
- 1 cup ice cubes

PREPARATION:

1. Add the peanut butter, cocoa powder, cream, chia seeds, vanilla extract, water, espresso powder, salt, and stevia to a blender and process until completely smooth.
2. Add the ice cubes and pulse until smooth.
3. Pour into a glass and enjoy immediately.

Lunch: Banana waffles (See page 71)

*Dinner: Cheese quesadillas (**See page 58**)*

DAY 15

Breakfast: Coconut pancakes
Time: 25 minutes | Serves 4
Carbohydrates: 3g/0.1oz | Fiber: 8g/0.3oz | Fat:24g/0.85oz
Protein: 12g/0.4oz | Calories: 290

INGREDIENTS:

- 6 eggs, separated
- ¾ cup coconut milk
- ½ cup coconut flour
- 2 tbsp melted coconut oil
- 1 tsp baking powder
- Pinch of salt
- Butter
- Berries for serving

PREPARATION:

1. Whip egg whites with salt in a bowl until it forms peaks.
2. Whisk yolks, coconut milk, and oil in a separate bowl. Add baking powder and coconut flour a little at a time and whisk to a smooth batter.
3. Fold in the egg whites, leave to thicken, then fry in a little butter on each side.
4. Serve with berries.

Lunch: Broccoli cheese soup (See page 41)

Dinner: Chicken korma (See page 56)

DAY 16

Breakfast: Blueberry smoothie (See page 76)

Lunch: Cobb salad
Time: 40 minutes | Serves 6
Carbohydrates: 10g/0.4oz | Fiber: 5g/0.2oz | Fat: 52g/1.83oz
Protein: 20g/0.8oz | Calories: 575

INGREDIENTS:

- ¼ cup red wine vinegar
- 2 tsp salt
- 1 tsp lemon juice
- 1l garlic clove, minced
- ¾ tsp pepper
- ¾ tsp Worcestershire sauce
- ¼ tsp sugar
- ¼ tsp ground mustard
- ¾ cup canola oil
- ¼ cup olive oil
- 6 ½ cups romaine
- 2 ½ cups curly endive
- 1 bunch watercress, trimmed
- 2 cooked chicken breasts, chopped
- 2 medium tomatoes, seeded and chopped
- 1 medium ripe avocado, peeled and chopped
- 3 hard-boiled large eggs, chopped
- ½ cup crumbled blue or Roquefort cheese
- 6 bacon strips, cooked and crumbled
- 2 tbsp chives, minced

PREPARATION:

1. Add the first 8 ingredients and process in a blender, adding a little canola and olive oil at a time.
2. Toss the romaine, endive and half the watercress in a bowl and transfer to plate.
3. Arrange the chicken, avocado, tomatoes, eggs, cheese, and bacon on top of the greens, sprinkle with chives and remaining watercress. Cover and refrigerate.
4. Drizzle the dressing over the salad and serve.

Dinner: Keto salmon pie (See page 54)

DAY 17

Breakfas: Crispy Prosciutto and Scallion Frittata (See page 30)

Lunch: Almond chicken salad
Time: 15 minutes | Serves 6
Carbohydrates: 10g/0.4oz | Fiber: 2g/0.08oz | Fat: 23g/0.81oz
Protein: 25g/0.82oz | Calories:351

INGREDIENTS:

- 4 cups cooked chicken, cubed
- 1½ cups green grapes, halved
- 1 cup celery, chopped
- ¾ cup sliced green onions
- 3 hard-boiled large eggs, chopped
- 1 1/2 cup Miracle Whip
- ¼ cup sour cream
- 1 tbsp prepared mustard
- 1 tsp salt
- ½ tsp pepper
- ¼ tsp onion powder
- ¼ tsp celery salt
- ⅛ tsp ground mustard
- ⅛ tsp paprika
- ½ cup almonds, toasted

PREPARATION:

1. Combine the first five ingredients in a large bowl and stir well.
2. Combine the following nine ingredients in a separate bowl and stir until smooth.
3. Add in the chicken mixture and toss.
4. Serve with sprinkled almonds on top.

Dinner: Basic low carb pizza (See page 53)

DAY 18

Breakfast: Blueberry smoothie (See page 76)

Lunch: Almond vegetable stir fry
Time: 20 minutes | Serves 5
Carbohydrates: 11g/0.4oz | Fiber: 3g/0.1oz | Fat: 10g/0.4oz
Protein: 4g/0.14oz | Calories:143

INGREDIENTS:

- 1 tsp cornstarch
- 1 tsp sugar
- 3 tbsp cold water
- 2 tbsp soy sauce
- 1 tsp sesame oil
- 4 cups broccoli florets
- 2 tbsp canola oil
- 1 large sweet red pepper, cut into 1-inch chunks
- 1 small onion, thinly sliced
- 2 garlic cloves, minced
- 1 tbsp minced fresh ginger root
- ¼ cup almonds, toasted

PREPARATION:

1. Combine cornstarch and sugar in a small bowl and stir in soy sauce, sesame oil, and water until smooth.
2. Stir-fry broccoli in a large wok on hgh for 3 minutes.
3. Add pepper, garlic, onion, and giner and stir-fry for 2 minutes.
4. Reduce heat then add soy sauce mixture and almonds, cooking for a further 2 minutes until thickened.

Dinner: Grilled chicken with spinach and melted mozzarella (See page 49)

DAY 19

Breakfast: Bulletproof coffee (See page 29)

Lunch: Veggie lasagna stuffed portobello mushrooms (See page 42)

Dinner: Mixed spice burgers
Time: 26 minutes | Serves 6
Carbohydrates: 2g/0.07oz | Fiber: 1g/0.03oz | Fat: 9g/0.3oz
Protein: 22g/0.8oz | Calories:192

INGREDIENTS:

- 1.5 lbs/680g ground beef
- 1 onion, finely chopped
- 1 clove garlic, minced
- 2 tbsp minced mint
- 3 tbsp minced parsley
- ¾ tsp pepper
- ¾ tsp ground allspice
- ½ tsp ground cinnamon
- ½ tsp salt
- ¼ ground nutmeg
- Lettuce leaves for serving

PREPARATION:

1. Add all the ingredients except beef to a bowl and mix.
2. Add in the ground beef and mix well.
3. Create 6 patties and fry each over a medium heat until cooked through.
4. Serve bunless with lettuce.

DAY 20

Breakfast: Green smoothie (See page 75)

Lunch: Broccoli cheese soup (See page 41)

Dinner: Garlic chicken
Time: 50 minutes | Serves 4
Carbohydrates: 3g/0.14oz | Fiber: 1g/0.03oz | Fat: 39g/1.4oz
Protein: 42g/1.5oz | Calories:546

INGREDIENTS:

- 2 lbs/900g chicken drumsticks
- 5 garlic cloves, sliced
- ½ cup finely chopped parsley
- 2 tbsp olive oil
- 4 tbsp butter
- Juice of one lemon

PREPARATION:

1. Preheat oven to 440°F/225°C.
2. Arrange drumsticks on a greased baking pan and top with salt, pepper, garlic, olie oil, parsley, and lemon juice.
3. Bake for 35-40 minutes or until golden brown.

DAY 21

Breakfast: Bulletproof coffee (See page 29)

Lunch: Kale stuffed portobello mushrooms (See page 40)

Dinner: Turnip fritters with bacon

Time: 20 minutes | Serves 4

Carbohydrates: 11g/0.4oz | Fiber: 7g/0.3oz | Fat: 92g/3.5oz

Protein: 24g/0.85oz | Calories: 978

INGREDIENTS:

- 4 eggs
- 15 oz/425g peeled and grated turnip
- 6oz/170g bacon
- 6oz/170g halloumi, grated
- 5oz/140g leafy greens
- 3oz/85g butter
- 1 cup mayonnaise
- 3 tbsp coconut flour
- 1 tsp salt
- ½ tsp onion powder
- ¼ tsp pepper
- ⅛ tsp turmeric

PREPARATION:

1. Combine all the ingredients except bacon, mayonnaise, and leafy greens in a bowl.
2. Create 12 patties and arrange in a frying pan, frying in butter a batch at a time.
3. Fry the bacon then serve with the patties, leafy greens, and mayonnaise.

DAY 22

Breakfast: Mushroom omelet (See page 31)

Lunch: Red pepper soup
Time: 55 minutes | Serves 12
Carbohydrates: 14g/0.5oz | Fiber: 2g/0.07oz | Fat: 2g/0.07oz
Protein: 2g/0.07oz | Calories:83

INGREDIENTS:

- 6 medium sweet red peppers, chopped
- 2 medium carrots, chopped
- 2 medium onions, chopped
- 1 celery, chopped
- 4 garlic cloves, minced
- 1 tbsp olive oil
- 64 oz/1.8l chicken stock
- ½ cup long grain rice
- 2 tbsp minced fresh thyme
- 1½ tsp salt
- ¼ tsp pepper
- ⅛ tsp cayenne pepper
- 11/8 tsp red pepper flakes

PREPARATION:

1. Add the red peppers, onions, carrots, celery, and garlic to a Dutch oven with a little oil and saute until tender.
2. Add in the stock, rice, thyme, salt, pepper, and cayenne and bring to a boil.
3. Reduce heat, cover, and simmer for 25 minutes until rice and veg are tender.
4. Remove from heat and cool for 30 minutes then puree ¼ at a time.
5. Return to pan, add red pepper flakes and warm through before serving.

Dinner: Eggplant Parmesan boats (See page 47)

DAY 23

Breakfast: Fried eggs with broiled tomatoes (See page 32)

Lunch: Blue cheese walnut tart
Time: 45 minutes | Serves 12
Carbohydrates: 10g/0.35oz | Fiber: 0g/0oz | Fat: 16g/0.56oz
Protein: 4g/0.014oz | Calories:197

INGREDIENTS:

- 1 sheet pie pastry
- 1 garlic clove, minced
- 1 egg
- 8 oz/225g cream cheese
- ⅓ cup crumbled blue cheese
- ¼ cup heavy whipping cream
- ¼ tsp cayenne pepper
- ¼ tsp coarsely ground pepper
- ⅓ cup chopped roasted sweet red peppers
- 3 tbsp chopped walnuts, toasted
- 2 tbsp minced fresh parsley

PREPARATION:

1. In an ungreased 9" tart pan with removable bottom, press pastry to create the tart. Trim any edges and bake for 10 minutes at 425°F/220°C.
2. Allow to cool on a wire rack.
3. Meanwhile, beat the cream cheese, blue cheese, and garlic in a large bowl.
4. Add the cream, egg, cayenne, and pepper and beat then spread mixture into the crust.
5. Sprinkle with peppers, walnuts, and parsley.
6. Bake at 375°F/190°C for 15-20 minutes or until centre has set.

Dinner: Shrimp scampi and spinach salad (See page 52)

DAY 24

Breakfast: Eggocado (See page 38)

Lunch: Curried chicken salad with pineapples and grapes
Time: 15 minutes | Serves 6
Carbohydrates: 14g/0.53oz | Fiber: 1g/0.03oz | Fat: 22g/0.77oz
Protein: 27g/0.95oz | Calories:364

INGREDIENTS:

- 4 cups cooked chicken, cubed
- 20 oz/566g pineapple chunks
- 1 cup seedless grapes, halved
- ½ cup mayonnaise
- ½ tsp curry powder

PREPARATION:

1. Add the chicken, pineapple, and grapes to a large bowl and mix.
2. In a separate bowl, add the mayonnaise and curry powder, pour over the chicken mixture, and toss to coat.
3. Serve fresh or keep refrigerated.

Dinner: Balsamic chicken with roast vegetables (See page 51)

DAY 25

Breakfast: Spinach and goat cheese frittata (See page 36)

Lunch: Eggplant Parmesan boats (See page 47)

Dinner: Zucchini pizza
Time: 40 minutes | Serves 6
Carbohydrates: 9g/0.3oz | Fiber: 1g/0.03oz | Fat: 12g/0.4oz
Protein: 14g/0.5oz | Calories:219

INGREDIENTS:

- 3 lightly beaten eggs
- 12oz/340g julienned roasted sweet peppers
- 2 cups shredded zucchini
- ½ cup grated Parmesan
- 1 cup shredded mozzarella cheese
- ½ cup sliced turkey pepperoni
- ¼ cup all purpose flour
- 1 tbsp minced thyme
- 1 tbsp olive oil
- 1 tbsp minced basil

PREPARATION:

1. Preheat oven to 450°F/220°C.
2. In a bowl, combine all ingredients except pepperoni and peppers.
3. Spread the mixture to a coated pizza pan.
4. Bake for 15 minutes.
5. Reduce temperature to 400°F/200°C and top with pepperoni and peppers.
6. Bake for a further 10 minutes and serve.

DAY 26

Breakfast: Coconut porridge (See page 37)

Lunch: Buffalo chicken lettuce wraps (See page 44)

Dinner: Chicken garam masala
Time: 25 minutes | Serves 4
Carbohydrates: 6g/0.2oz | Fiber: 4g/0.1oz | Fat: 51g/1.8oz
Protein: 38g/1.34oz | Calories:620

INGREDIENTS:

- 25oz/700g chicken breasts, cut lengthwise
- 1¼ cups coconut cream
- 1 finely chopped red bell pepper
- 3 tbsp butter
- 2½ tbsp sugar-free garam masala
- 1 tbsp finely chopped parsley
- Salt

PREPARATION:

1. Preheat oven to 400°F/200°C.
2. Fry chicken in butter over a medium high heat.
3. Add half the garam masala, place on a baking dish and sprinkle with salt and juices from the pan.
4. In a small bowl, mix the bell pepper, coconut cream, and remaining garam masala.
5. Add to the chicken and bake for 22 minutes.
6. Serve with parsley.

DAY 27

Breakfast: Spinach and goat cheese frittata (See page 36)

Lunch: Broccoli cheese soup (See page 41)

Dinner: Tuna casserole
Time: 30 minutes | Serves 4
Carbohydrates: 5g/0.18oz | Fiber: 3g/0.1oz | Fat: 83g/3oz
Protein: 43g/1.5oz | Calories:953

INGREDIENTS:

- 15oz/425g tin of tuna
- 6oz/170g baby spinach
- 5oz/140g finely chopped celery stalks
- 2oz/57g butter
- 1 finely chopped yellow onion
- 4oz/114g shredded parmesan cheese
- 1 finely chopped green bell pepper
- 4 tbsp olive oil
- 1 cup mayonnaise
- 1 tsp chili flakes
- Salt and pepper

PREPARATION:

1. Preheat oven to 400°F/200°C.
2. Fry pepper, onion, and celery in butter and season.
3. Transfer to a greased baking dish and add the tuna, mayonnaise, cheese, and chilli flakes and bake until golden brown.
4. Serve with baby spinach and olive oil.

DAY 28

Breakfast: Bulletproof coffee (See page 29)

Lunch: Kale stuffed portobello mushrooms (See page 40)

Dinner: Chicken provençale
Time: 70 minutes | Serves 4
Carbohydrates: 5g/0.18oz | Fiber: 3g/0.1oz | Fat: 78g/2.75oz
Protein: 43g/1.5oz | Calories:911

INGREDIENTS:

- 2lbs/900g chicken thighs
- 7oz/200g lettuce
- 8oz/225g tomatoes
- 5 sliced garlic cloves
- 1 cup mayonnaise
- ¼ cup olive oil
- ½ cup pitted black olives
- 1 tbsp dried oregano
- 1 tsp paprika powder
- Zest of ¼ lemon
- Salt and pepper

PREPARATION:

1. Preheat oven to 400°F/200°C.
2. Add the chicken to an ovenproof baking dish and place garlic, olives, and tomatoes around it. Sprinkle over oregano, salt, pepper, and a drizzle of olive oil.
3. Roast for an hour until cooked through.
4. Mix mayonnaise, lemon zest, paprika powder, salt, and pepper for dressing.
5. Serve chicken with dressing, roasted veggies, and lettuce.

Printed in Great Britain
by Amazon

45331029R00063